The Adapt Program

A Low Carbohydrate, Ketogenic Diet Manual

By Dr. Eric C. Westman, MD MHS

Medical Disclaimer

The material in this book is for informational purposes only and is not intended as a substitute for the advice and care of your physician. Any new lifestyle program as outlined in this book should be followed only after first consulting with your physician to make sure it is appropriate for your individual circumstance.

The author and its publisher disclaim responsibility for any adverse effects that may result from the use or application of the information contained in this manual.

© 2015 Adapt Your Life Inc.

Preface

The Adapt Program way of eating has been around for awhile—it was first described in 1863 by William Banting. Because the body burns what it is fed, when you eliminate carbohydrates from the food, the body is forced to start burning fat--including its own stored fat. In England, up until the 1950s, if you wanted to lose weight you were told to do the Banting Diet-- a type of low carbohydrate diet.

Lost from the medical/nutritional world for 50 years, but carried on by a few clinical doctors, low carb diets are making a comeback because the scientific community started to re-evaluate these diets for safety. (There were no published studies about low carbohydrate diets for twenty years: from 1980-2002.) Now, many studies show that the low carbohydrate, high fat Adapt Program way of eating is healthy, and therapeutic for many chronic medical conditions like diabetes, pre-diabetes, metabolic syndrome and obesity.

Recent research suggests that when your body burns fat for its primary fuel, the body runs more efficiently and has less "wear and tear" from inflammation and oxidative stress. Even more exciting is the potential that this way of eating may be useful to optimize physical performance and to prevent or treat conditions like cancer and Alzheimer's Disease.

The science has come a long way since our first paper was published in 2002, ending a 20+ year taboo against studying low carbohydrate diets. I feel privileged to have been part of that research and also privileged to be able to provide this information to you today.

Dr. Eric C. Westman, MD MHS
Adapt Your Life Inc.

Adapt Program: Getting Started

List of Permitted Foods
To be most effective, keep the dietary carbohydrate to **less than 20 total carbs per day**. Stay to the foods on this list! It doesn't matter how the food is cooked. Make sure that there is no starchy breading or sauce on the food.

When hungry, EAT AS MUCH AS YOU WANT OF THE FOLLOWING FOODS. (These foods have no carbs.)
Meat: Beef (hamburger, steak), pork, ham, bacon, lamb, veal, sausage, pepperoni, hot dogs, organ meats like liver, kidney, and sweetbreads.
Poultry: Chicken, turkey, duck, pheasant or other fowl.
Fish & Shellfish: Any fish including tuna, salmon, catfish, bass, trout, shrimp, scallops, crab, and lobster.
Eggs: Whole eggs (whites and yolks).

Don't avoid the fat. You do not have to deliberately limit quantities of these foods, but stop eating when full.

Salad Greens and Nonstarchy Vegetables should be eaten every day, but the amount is limited:
Salad Greens: 2 cups a day. Includes: arugula, bok choy, cabbage, chard, chives, endive, greens (beet, collards, mustard, and turnip), kale, lettuce, parsley, spinach, radicchio, radishes, scallions, and watercress.

Nonstarchy Vegetables: 1 cup a day. Includes: artichokes, asparagus, broccoli, Brussel sprouts, cauliflower, celery, cucumber, dikon, eggplant, green beans (string beans), jicama, leeks, mushrooms, okra, onions, peppers, pumpkin, rhubarb, shallots, snow peas, sprouts (bean & alfalfa) sugar-snap peas, summer squash, tomatoes, wax beans, zucchini.

If you do not have high blood pressure (hypertension) or heart failure, then use bouillon AS NEEDED during the first few weeks to minimize headache or fatigue.
***Bouillon:** up to 2 times daily.* Clear broth (consommé) can be used as well. Unless you are told to restrict your salt intake, there is no need to use low sodium bouillon.

FOODS THAT ARE ALLOWED IN LIMITED QUANTITIES:
(Check the labels to be sure there are no added carbs.)
***Oils:** 2 tablespoonfuls a day.* Includes: butter, coconut oil, peanut oil, palm oil. Avoid seed oils.
Cheese: up to 4 ounces a day. Includes: hard, aged cheeses such as swiss, cheddar, brie, camembert, bleu, mozzarella, gruyere, cream cheese, goat cheeses.
Cream: up to 2 tablespoonfuls a day. Includes whipping, heavy, light, sour cream, half and half.
Mayonnaise: *up to 2 tablespoons a day.*
Olives (black or green): up to 6 a day.
***Avocado:** up to ½ of a fruit a day.*
Lemon/lime juice: up to 2 teaspoonfuls a day.
***Soy sauces:** up to 2 tablespoons a day.*
Pickles, dill or sugar-free: *up to 2 serving a day.*
Adapt Products: up to 2 servings per day.

Zero Carb Snacks: Sugar-free jello, pork rinds (chicarrones); "roll-up" (cheese wrapped in slice of meat) boerewors, biltong, beef jerky, deviled eggs

Limiting carbs leads to fat burning, but it doesn't always mean you will lose fat weight. Fat loss occurs when you are eating fewer calories than you are burning. On the Adapt Program, the reduction in hunger should lead to an automatic reduction in the amount that you eat.

How It Works
The Adapt Program way of eating changes the fuel that your body uses from mainly carbohydrate (sugars and starches) to mainly fat. Your body is turned into a "fat burning machine." Being a fat burning machine is a good way to use up your stored body fat (to lose fat weight).

Science tells up that an elevated blood sugar (glucose) is the pathway toward obesity and diabetes, and it is the hormone insulin that tells the body to make fat and to store fat. Because insulin is secreted in response to an elevated blood sugar, a simple way to keep insulin low is by *eating* foods that don't raise the blood sugar (fat and protein), and by *not eating* foods that raise the blood sugar (carbohydrate).

When you eat the Adapt Your Life way, your body will be provided the nutrition that it needs and the fuel that your body uses will be changed from mainly carbohydrate to mainly fat. The Adapt Program way of eating is particularly good if you are trying to control the blood sugar, reduce body fat, or enhance blood ketones.

How Many Carbohydrates?
One way to measure the amount of sugars and starches in the diet is by counting "carbohydrate grams" or "carbs." To increase your body's fat burning, we recommend that your carb intake be less than 20 grams per day. When you eat even a small amount of carbs, you reduce your body's ability to burn fat. This means that you will need to avoid sugar (5 grams/teaspoon), bread (15 grams/slice), fruit (20 grams/apple), flour, pasta, or any other food that has a lot of carbohydrates. A list of the foods initially allowed is provided to assist you in changing your eating habits. What you will notice is that your hunger will go away in just a day or two.

Because you are less hungry, you will eat less and start burning your own body fat, which leads to weight loss.

If you are not in good health, or if you are taking medications, medical supervision by someone trained in this type of program is highly recommended. As your weight decreases and your medical conditions improve, the medications that you are taking will probably have to be reduced. There are also certain blood tests that should be checked periodically to make sure that your values are within the normal range. Many people say that it is helpful to have regularly-scheduled appointments to ensure that they follow the diet by providing "accountability."

Possible Side Effects

Changing to this new way or eating may have some side effects during the first week. Some people experience sugar cravings, fatigue, headaches, body aches, difficulty concentrating, or other flu-like symptoms. These symptoms are usually mild and pass quickly, and are a sign that your body is going through a transition period from burning carbohydrates to burning fat for fuel. To avoid or minimize these side effects:

Drink Lots of Liquids: It is important to drink an adequate amount of fluid per day – preferably water or another non-caffeinated beverage. Drink when thirsty.

Drink Bouillon or Broth: If you do not have high blood pressure or heart failure, drink bouillon or broth one to three times a day. To make the broth, drop a cube of bouillon into a cup of hot water and drink it. Although your energy levels will soon return to normal, many patients have reported they enjoy the broth and continue drinking it beyond the first week.

Sugar cravings: You may initially experience cravings for the sugary/starch foods that you used to eat, but the cravings will pass in a few days. Sugar cravings can be temporarily treated with a sugar-free beverage, such as diet soda, or a sugar-free flavoring, or sugar-free jello with whipped cream.

Breath: Rarely, some people experience bad breath in the initial stages changing to this way of eating. This can usually be avoided by drinking plenty of water and performing good oral hygiene (seeing a dentist, brushing your teeth twice a day (including your tongue), and flossing your teeth daily). Sugar-free gum or mints may also be helpful.

Constipation: Most people notice they have to go to the bathroom less often to have a bowel movement. How often you have a bowel movement is not a medical issue. But, if you are experiencing hard stools or hard-to-pass stools, this is called constipation, and there are a number of ways to address this issue.
- use 1 teaspoon of milk of magnesia at bedtime daily
- add ½ cup of fiber-rich vegetables to your diet per day
- have 1 to 2 servings per day of sugar-free gum or sugar-free candy that contains sugar alcohols
- use sugar-free fiber supplement twice a day

If the issue persists, consult your health care provider.

Ketosis: Ketosis is okay, it means that your body is burning fat, and that's a good thing. (Ketosis is commonly confused with 'ketoacidosis'- a serious condition that can occur in individuals with diabetes.) You can measure your urine or blood or breath ketones at home if you want, but that is not needed for most people.

What happens if I "slip"?: Once you begin this way of eating, you must follow it strictly. If you eat carbohydrates, even a little bit, you may stop the weight loss process for up to three days. This means you will come out of ketosis (fat-burning), and you may even gain back several pounds of water weight. The most important thing to do if you "slip" and eat carbohydrates is to get right back on track with the next meal. You'll be surprised that it is not difficult to be strict because your hunger will be decreased or gone entirely.

Vitamins and Supplements: Although this way of eating is very nutritious, we recommend that you take an iron-free multivitamin to be sure that you are getting all of the vitamins and minerals that you need.

Cholesterol: Many people ask how this way of eating will affect blood cholesterol levels and risk for heart disease. Many people were taught that this way of eating was unhealthy because it is high in fat. The predictions about how this way of eating would adversely affect the blood cholesterol didn't come true when the studies were finally done. This way of eating reduces the cardiac risk factors by lowering blood triglycerides and increasing the good cholesterol (HDL).

More Than Weight Loss: If you have excess weight, and you adhere to your new way of eating, you can expect to lose pounds and inches. Most people also have improved energy levels, better appetite control, and a reduction in symptoms of many health problems you may have experienced before. If you have diabetes, you can expect better blood sugar control and a reduction in your diabetes medications may have to be made on the day you stop eating carbohydrates. However, if you are taking diabetes medications, including insulin, do not change the dosage or stop taking without consulting with your health care provider.

Increasing Activity and Reducing Stress: Increasing your activity level may help reduce stress, decrease appetite, build muscle, and improve bone density.
Stress management techniques may improve your ability to handle dietary temptations, sugar cravings, and emotional eating patterns.

The Main Restriction: Carbohydrates
The main restriction is that no sugars (simple carbohydrates) and no starches (complex carbohydrates) are eaten. The only carbohydrates we encourage are the nutritionally-dense, fiber rich vegetables listed on page 4 and 5.

Sugars are simple carbohydrates. **Avoid these kinds of foods**: white sugar, brown sugar, honey, maple syrup, molasses, corn syrup, beer (contains barley malt), milk (contains lactose), flavored yogurts, fruit juice, and fruit.

Starches are complex carbohydrates. **Avoid these kinds of foods**: grains (even "whole" grains), rice, cereals, flour, cornstarch, breads, pastas, muffins, bagels, crackers, and "starchy" vegetables such as slow-cooked beans (pinto, lima, black beans, etc.), carrots, parsnips, corn, peas, potatoes, French fries, potato chips, etc.

Fats and Oils
All fats and oils, even butter, are allowed. Olive oil and peanut oil are especially healthy oils and are encouraged in cooking. Avoid margarine and other hydrogenated oils.

For salad dressings, use oil and vinegar, bleu cheese, ranch, Caesar, Italian. Avoid "lite" dressings, as these commonly have more carbohydrate. Chopped eggs, bacon, and/or grated cheese may also be included in salads.

Fats, in general, are important to include because they taste good and make you feel full. You, therefore, can eat the fat or skin that is served with the meat or poultry that you eat, as long as there is no breading on the skin. **Do not attempt to follow a low-fat diet! It makes no sense when your body is burning fat for its primary fuel.**

Sweeteners and Desserts
You can have sweet things to eat and drink, just not things sweetened with sugar. Some available alternative sweeteners are: Splenda (sucralose), Nutrasweet (aspartame), Truvia (stevia/erythritol blend), Sweet & Low (saccharin), sugar alcohols (sorbitol, maltitol). Sugar alcohols can occasionally cause stomach upset.

Beverages
Drink as much as you would like of the allowed beverages, but do not force fluids beyond your capacity. The best beverage is water.

Caffeinated beverages: Some patients find that their caffeine intake interferes with their weight loss and blood sugar control. With this in mind, you may have **up to 3 servings** of coffee (black, or with artificial sweetener and/or cream), tea (unsweetened or artificially sweetened), or caffeinated diet soda per day.

Alcohol
At first, we ask that you avoid alcohol consumption. As weight loss and dietary patterns become well-established, alcohol in moderate quantities may be added back at a later point in time. We can help you make the best choices for low-carbohydrate alcoholic beverages if needed.

Quantities
Eat when you are hungry; stop when you are full. Learn to listen to your body. A low-carbohydrate diet has a natural appetite reduction effect to ease you into the consumption of smaller and smaller quantities comfortably. If you are not hungry, you don't have to eat. You do not have to eat everything on your plate "just because it's there." You are not counting calories.

Important Reminders
If the food is not on Page 4 and 5--you can't have it!

Avoid these common mistakes: Beware of "fat-free" or "lite" diet products and foods containing "hidden" sugars and starches (such as coleslaw or sugar-free cookies and cakes). Check the labels of liquid medications, cough syrups, cough drops, and other over-the-counter medications that may contain sugar. Avoid products that are labeled "Great for Low-Carb Diets!" If you are counting Total Carbs (which I recommend at first), then ignore "Net Carb" calculations.

Adapt Products
If you are using low carbohydrate products, look for the Adapt Products (www.adaptyourlife.com).

Adapt Program Menu Planning

What does a low-carb menu look like? You can plan your daily menu by using the following as a guide:

Breakfast
Meat or other protein source (usually eggs)
Fat source -- *This may already be in your protein, for example, bacon & eggs have fat in them.*
Low-carb vegetable (if desired) – *This can be in an omelet or breakfast quiche.*

Lunch
Meat or other protein source
Fat source -- *butter, salad dressing, cheese, cream, avocado, etc.*
1 to 1 ½ cups of salad greens or cooked greens
½ to 1 cup of vegetables

Snack
Low-carb snack that has protein and/or fat

Dinner
Meat or other protein source
Fat source -- *If your protein is "lean"—add some fat with butter, salad dressing, cheese, cream, avocado, etc.*
1 to 1 ½ cups of salad greens or cooked greens
½ to 1 cup of vegetables

A Sample Day of the Adapt Program

Breakfast
Eggs, any style
Bacon or sausage

Lunch
Grilled chicken salad with full fat salad dressing

Snack
Pepperoni slices and a cheese stick
Adapt Product

Dinner
Burger patty or steak
Green salad with other vegetables and salad dressing
Green beans with butter

Reading a Nutrition Facts Label: United States Labelling

There are two ways to count carbs: TOTAL CARBS or NET CARBS
- _X_ Use TOTAL CARBS
    - Look only at Total Carbohydrate
    - In the example below, the total carbohydrate is 19 grams per serving
    - Look at serving size
    - TOTAL CARBS are used in clinics using the low carbohydrate ketogenic diet, and by the Adapt Your Life Program

- NET CARBS
    - Subtract fiber and artificial sweeteners from the total carbohydrate to get the "net carb grams"
    - In the example below, 19 grams carbohydrate – 2 grams fiber = 17 grams of net carbs per serving
    - Look at serving size
    - NET CARBS are used in generally healthy individuals

Also check the ingredient list. Avoid foods that have any form of sugar or starch listed in the first 5 ingredients.

Reading a Nutrition Facts Label: United States Labelling

Nutrition Facts	
Serving Size (117g)	
Servings Per Container 1	
Amount Per Serving	
Calories 160	Calories from Fat 70
	% Daily Value*
Total Fat 8g	12%
Saturated Fat 3g	15%
Trans Fat 0g	
Cholesterol 0mg	0%
Sodium 5mg	0%
Total Carbohydrate 19g	6%
Dietary Fiber 2g	8%
Sugars 14g	
Protein 2g	
Vitamin A 2% • Vitamin C 8%	
Calcium 2% • Iron 2%	

*Percent Daily Values are based on a 2,000 calorie diet. Your daily values may be higher or lower depending on your calorie needs:

		Calories:	2,000	2,500
Total Fat	Less than		65g	80g
Saturated Fat	Less than		20g	25g
Cholesterol	Less than		300mg	300mg
Sodium	Less than		2,400mg	2,400mg
Total Carbohydrate			300g	375g
Dietary Fiber			25g	30g

Calories per gram:
   Fat 9 • Carbohydrate 4 • Protein 4

This product has 19 grams of Total Carbs. In the U.S., the Total Carbohydrate calculation includes the fiber content.

To obtain the Net Carbs, subtract the 2 grams of fiber from the total carbohydrate. So, Net Carbs is 19 - 2 = 17 grams.

Reading a Nutrition Facts Label: Outside U.S.A.

There are two ways to count carbs: TOTAL CARBS or NET CARBS
- _X_ Use TOTAL CARBS
    - Look at Total Carbohydrate
    - Add fiber grams to total carbohydrate grams
    - In the example below, the total carbohydrate is 17 grams + 2 grams of fiber = 19 grams per serving
    - Look at serving size
    - TOTAL CARBS are used in clinics using the low carbohydrate ketogenic diet, and by the Adapt Your Life Program

- NET CARBS
    - Outside the U.S.A. the total carbohydrate (or glycaemic carbohydrate) number represents Net Carbs, because the fiber grams are already subtracted
    - In the example below, the Net Carbs is 17 grams per serving
    - Look at serving size
    - NET CARBS are used in generally healthy individuals

Also check the ingredient list. Avoid foods that have any form of sugar or starch listed in the first 5 ingredients.

Reading a Nutrition Facts Label: Outside U.S.A.

Nutrition Information	Per 100 g	Per portion of 117 g %Reference Intake RI
Energy	504 kJ / 121 kcal	638 kJ / 153 kcal 8% RI
Fat	6 g	8 g 11% RI
Of which Saturates	2,5 g	2,9 g 15% RI
Carbohydrate	14 g	17 g 7% RI
Of which Sugars	12 g	14 g 16% RI
Protein	1,6 g	1,9 g 4% RI
Salt content is exclusively due to the presence of naturally occurring sodium.		
Contains negligible amounts of Salt.		
Reference intake of an average adult (8 400 kJ / 2 000 kcal)		

Due to the method of calculation, the "Total Carbohdyrate" or "Glycaemic Carbohydrate" on the nutrition facts label already has the fiber grams subtracted from the number.

So, "Total Carbohydrate" outside the U.S.A. is the same as "Net Carbohydrate" within the U.S.A.

Outside the U.S.A., to obtain the Total Carbohydrate content, add the fiber grams to the total grams.

Adapt Program Reminders

"Carbs make you hungry"

"Fruit makes you fat"

"Fruit is nature's candy"

"There is only one teaspoon of sugar in the human bloodstream"

"Nothing tastes as good as thin feels"

"Eat fat to burn fat"

"Don't fear the fat"

"It makes sense to eat fat when your body is a fat-burning machine"

"There are two ways to feel full: stretch the stomach or eat fat"

"Corn is fed to animals to make fatty liver (foie gras) and to fatten them up"

"It's not YOUR fault—it's the carbs' fault"

"You don't have to eat everything on your plate!"

"Eat when hungry, drink when thirsty"

Date	Weight	Waistline
_____	_____	_____
_____	_____	_____
_____	_____	_____
_____	_____	_____
_____	_____	_____
_____	_____	_____
_____	_____	_____
_____	_____	_____
_____	_____	_____
_____	_____	_____
_____	_____	_____
_____	_____	_____
_____	_____	_____
_____	_____	_____
_____	_____	_____
_____	_____	_____

Date	Weight	Waistline
_____	_____	_____
_____	_____	_____
_____	_____	_____
_____	_____	_____
_____	_____	_____
_____	_____	_____
_____	_____	_____
_____	_____	_____
_____	_____	_____
_____	_____	_____
_____	_____	_____
_____	_____	_____
_____	_____	_____
_____	_____	_____
_____	_____	_____
_____	_____	_____

Date	Weight	Waistline
_____	_____	_____
_____	_____	_____
_____	_____	_____
_____	_____	_____
_____	_____	_____
_____	_____	_____
_____	_____	_____
_____	_____	_____
_____	_____	_____
_____	_____	_____
_____	_____	_____
_____	_____	_____
_____	_____	_____
_____	_____	_____
_____	_____	_____
_____	_____	_____
_____	_____	_____

Date	Weight	Waistline
_____	_____	_____
_____	_____	_____
_____	_____	_____
_____	_____	_____
_____	_____	_____
_____	_____	_____
_____	_____	_____
_____	_____	_____
_____	_____	_____
_____	_____	_____
_____	_____	_____
_____	_____	_____
_____	_____	_____
_____	_____	_____
_____	_____	_____

Date	Weight	Waistline
_____	_____	_____
_____	_____	_____
_____	_____	_____
_____	_____	_____
_____	_____	_____
_____	_____	_____
_____	_____	_____
_____	_____	_____
_____	_____	_____
_____	_____	_____
_____	_____	_____
_____	_____	_____
_____	_____	_____
_____	_____	_____
_____	_____	_____
_____	_____	_____

Notes

Notes

Contact Information

It is important to us that you feel comfortable contacting us about any issues you may have. Please use the following information to keep in touch:

Clinic name or practitioner:

_____

_____

Clinic phone:

_____

Email:

_____

Printed in Great Britain
by Amazon